a morning cup of
balance™

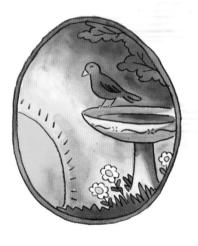

SWEET
WATER
PRESS

This edition published for Sweetwater Press by arrangement with
Crane Hill Publishers.

ISBN 1-58173-531-6

Book design by Miles G. Parsons
Illustrations by Tim Rocks
Cover art by Christena Brooks and Tim Rocks

Printed in China

a morning cup of
balance
™

one 15-minute routine for a lifetime of strength & stability

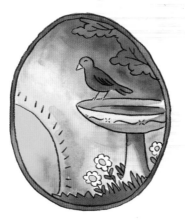

kim bright-fey, p.t.

SWEET WATER PRESS

Acknowledgments

Thank you to all of my patients, clients, and students
for providing constant inspiration.

Thank you to all at Crane Hill Publishers for showing an
interest in this work and making it become a reality.

To John, my husband,
who taught me the meaning of balance, the importance of
awareness, and the power in seeing myself as a teacher.

He also taught me the New Forest® Way. It has made me
a better physical therapist, a better person.

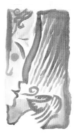

Contents

Foreword 7

Why Do I Need Balance? 8

Balance and Life 11
    Your Environment and Balance 13
    Your Body and Balance 13
    Risk Factor Checklist 14
    Your Balance System 16
    The Secret to Good Balance 17
    Test Your Balance 20

The Balance Routine 23

Getting the Most from Your Balance Routine 61
    Using Imagery for Better Balance 62
    A Sip of Tai Chi for Balance 69

Tips for Preventing Falls 75

Routine at a Glance 79

Foreword

Standing upright brings with it the challenge of maintaining an inherently unstable posture, particularly as we age. In *A Morning Cup of Balance*, Kim Bright-Fey has outlined a set of easy and enjoyable activities that help maintain posture and protect from potentially serious falls through the improvement of balance.

Research has shown that any exercise that helps build muscular strength and endurance will improve your ability to function in your daily life. If we maintain our strength, we are more active, more independent, and more interesting people, and can lead more interesting and fulfilling lives. I recommend the program in *A Morning Cup of Balance* as a simple and effective means to achieve this.

Dr. Alan Walmsley
Institute of Food, Nutrition, and Human Health
Massey University, Wellington, New Zealand

Dr. Alan Walmsley is an expert in Sport & Exercise Science, Biomechanics, and Ergonomics. He conducts research in the areas of Physical Performance, Fitness Assessment, Exercise Prescription, and Fall Prevention in the Elderly.

Why Do I Need Balance?

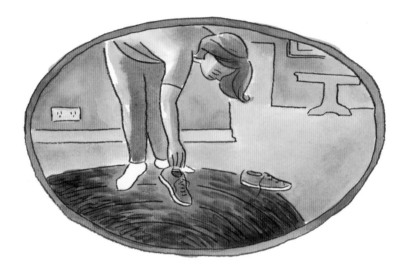

Every move you make requires balance. Reaching into the cupboard for your morning cup, picking up your shoe from the floor, and stepping out of the tub all depend on your body's ability to orchestrate a complex series of events. Playing golf, tennis, even walking the dog, requires balance. The more challenging the movement, the more balance you need.

I've been teaching exercises that improve balance, build strength and flexibility, and reduce stress for almost twenty years. Within the last decade, my work has become focused on preventing illness and injury. As a health and wellness specialist, I consider balance training to be the most important aspect of any fitness program.

Better balance gives you a better life. It is a key component to aging successfully and preventing injuries like sprained ankles and broken hips, particularly from falls. For millions of Americans, falls present a serious health risk. One out of every three adults age sixty-five and older falls each year, and falls are a leading cause of accidental death.

Studies show that millions of people live in fear of falling and fear that they will end up in a nursing home. It is a documented fact that the thought of falling and sustaining an injury can be more debilitating than actually falling. More and more people are spending their days at home, sitting in a chair, limiting their activity and social interactions in an effort to stay safe and avoid falling.

The statistics are frightening, but you don't need to be afraid of falling. My goal is to share with you the benefits of my experience. I offer my expertise as a physical therapist combined with my training in Tai Chi, the best-known balance exercise, to give you the opportunity to learn about your balance and improve it, in the comfort of your own home, without any fancy equipment.

You CAN improve your balance. This book will show you how. If you are like me, you probably feel tempted to start the exercise routine right away. Please, take my advice and read the opening material first. Understanding how balance works before starting the exercise routine will give you the best results.

It is time to take a sip from *A Morning Cup of Balance*. Within a week or two, you will be able to complete the series of exercises in about 15 minutes, and you should notice a big improvement in your balance.

Kim Bright-Fey
Birmingham, Alabama
Fall 2005

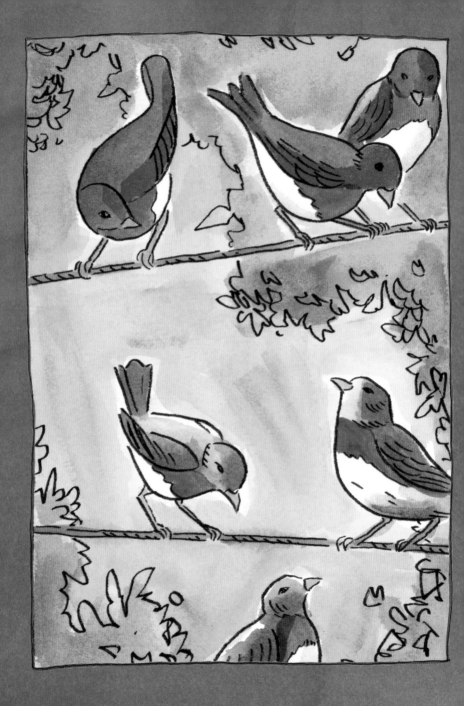

Balance and Life

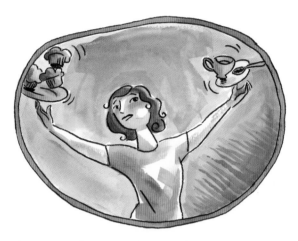

Every day you perform a multitude of balancing acts. You juggle your responsibilities at home and at work. You manage your income and expenses. You experience joy from the accomplishments of ones you love and frustration from waiting in line at the bank.

Maintaining a balanced life requires flexibility. You can't get hung up on any one thing. It requires strength. You must stay focused and determined to accomplish your goals and daily responsibilities. Most importantly, a balanced life requires perspective. Your thoughts and your attitude determine your ability to maintain a balanced life.

A balanced body is not much different. It requires flexibility, to allow movement in any direction. It requires strength, to stabilize and hold a position. And it requires perspective—an awareness and ability to process the information coming to your brain from your eyes, skin, muscles, and joints.

Good balance is necessary for a healthy, active, and independent lifestyle!

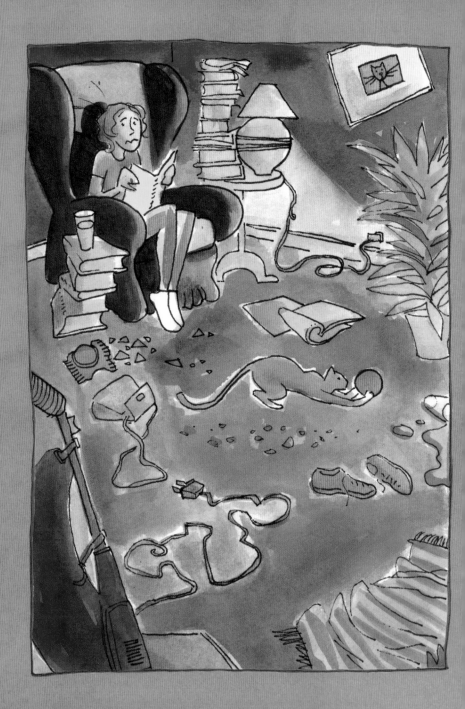

Your Environment and Balance

Take a look around. Do you see anything that might affect your ability to balance?

Floors cluttered with books, toys, or even too much furniture can turn any room into an obstacle course! Losing your balance happens in a split second. As they say, an ounce of prevention is worth a pound of cure. Take the time to make your home environment safe.

- Keep your floors and walkways clutter-free.
- Get rid of throw rugs that slide around or clump up.
- Install adequate lighting indoors and out.
- Use nightlights.
- Have flashlights available for power outages.
- Get rid of wobbly furniture.
- Install steady handrails on staircases and grab bars by the tub and shower.

Your Body and Balance

Any condition that affects your strength, flexibility, body (sensory) awareness, endurance, or cognition can have a negative effect on your balance. A decrease in your ability to balance can increase your risk of sustaining an injury. Identifying conditions that can impair your balance will help you identify your level of risk.

Risk Factor Checklist

Take a minute to look over the list of risk factors on the next page. Check the ones that apply to you.

If you checked more than one condition, you might have a higher risk of sustaining a balance-related injury. It is always a good idea to talk to your doctor before starting any exercise program. This is especially true before starting a balance-training program.

Sometimes, you need more than just exercise to improve your balance. Your doctor may need to review your medications, or refer you to a balance specialist like a physical therapist.

Dedicating fifteen minutes a day to the balance routine in this book is a great way to take control of your balance ability. The balance-training exercises in this book will:

- Improve your strength and flexibility
- Improve your body awareness
- Improve your focus and concentration

You will FEEL stronger, more flexible, and more confident!

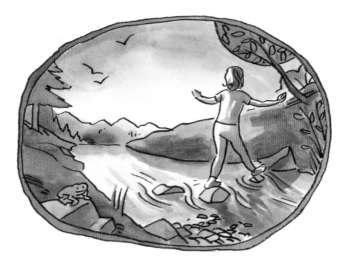

Risk Factor Checklist

Do you have any of these conditions?

❑	Impaired vision
❑	Impaired hearing
❑	Neuropathy or numbness
❑	Vertigo or dizziness
❑	Paralysis/nerve damage
❑	Arthritis or chronic pain condition
❑	Joint replacement: hip, knee, or shoulder
❑	Old injury: like ankle sprain or knee injury
❑	Back or neck pain
❑	Heart disease
❑	Poor circulation: cold hands and feet
❑	Lung problems
❑	Poor sleep patterns
❑	Take 4 or more medications each day
❑	Problems with attention
❑	Problems with memory
❑	Sedentary lifestyle
❑	Age 50 or older

Your Balance System

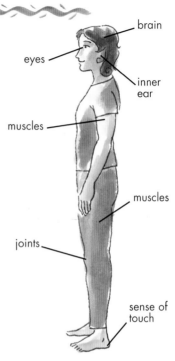

Your ability to maintain balance depends on multiple body systems.

Eyes/Vision

Your vision anchors you to your surroundings. What you see helps you determine the position of your body and guides your movement choices. Vision allows you to avoid obstacles and slippery floors. Try standing with your eyes closed to discover how much you use your vision to help you keep your balance.

Inner Ear/Vestibular System

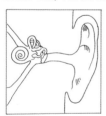

Your inner ear contains a very tiny but very sophisticated sensing and positioning device. This system sends signals to your brain to relay the position of your head. When your eyes are closed, your vestibular system can tell you if your body is horizontal, vertical, or tilted.

Kinesthetic Awareness

Kinesthetic (kin-is-thet-ic) awareness is a big term that describes the sensing ability of your entire body. Your skin has pressure receptors. You feel pressure on the bottoms of your feet when you are standing. Deep inside your muscles and joints, you have tiny proprioceptors (pro-pree-o-septors) that tell you the position of your arms and legs. You know when your hand is open or closed without looking. The receptors or sensing devices in your skin, muscles, and joints provide valuable information about the limitations of your body and help you keep your balance.

The Secret to Good Balance

I sincerely believe that the secret to good balance is body awareness. Balance is accomplished primarily on a subconscious level. Most of the time, you don't think about keeping your balance—you just do! As you grow older, thinking about your balance becomes more and more frequent. What came naturally in your youth now takes a bit more effort and concentration.

Bringing balance to a conscious level requires learning how to tune in to your body listening skills. I like to compare it to the volume knob on your radio. Your body is constantly sending you information. If you are like most people, you probably only hear the strongest, loudest signals. Most likely, you ignore your aches and pains until the signal gets so loud that you can't ignore it any longer.

Good balance depends on your ability to hear the quiet, early warning signals. To improve your balance, you need to have a sense of how your balance is right now. You need to have awareness of your body—how it feels and how it moves. You need to discover your limits of stability. In other words, what is the size of your balance safety zone?

Your balance safety zone is like a bubble that surrounds you. If you have poor balance, your safety zone is small. You keep your movements close to your body. You don't like to reach very high or very far away from yourself. You walk with short quick steps and you don't like to be distracted. Your daily routine is predictable. It makes you nervous to go to new or crowded places.

If you have good balance, your safety zone is large. You confidently move in any direction and are not afraid to reach for

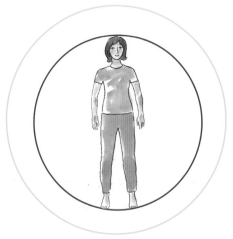

that cup on the top shelf. You walk with long strides, carrying bags of groceries and talking on the phone. You like to try new things and go to new places.

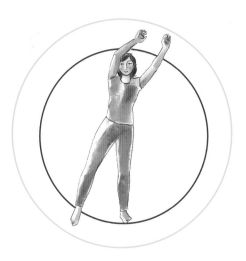

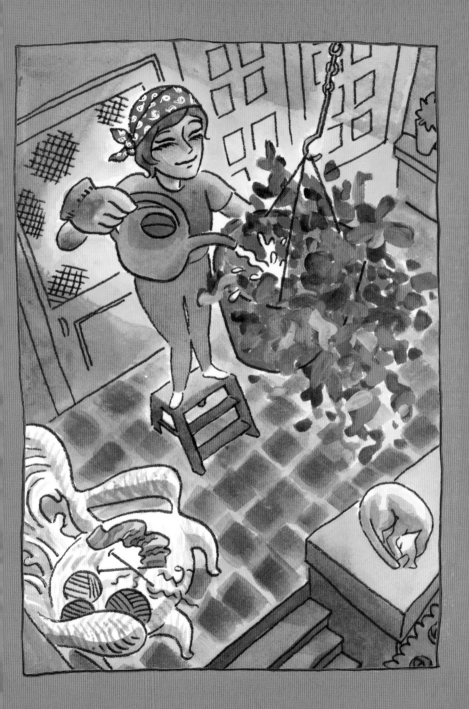

Test Your Balance ~~~~~~

Before you begin your morning cup routine, do this simple test to assess how your balance is today. Record your results and retest yourself in one month. Circle the choice below that applies.

Sit on a firm chair. Without using your hands, slowly come to a standing position.

This was: Easy   Slightly Challenging   Hard

Without moving your feet, reach forward 10 inches.

This was: Easy   Slightly Challenging   Hard

Stand 30 seconds with feet together and eyes closed.

This was: Easy   Slightly Challenging   Hard

Stand 20 seconds on one leg.

This was: Easy   Slightly Challenging   Hard

In slow motion, lift your knee and take a step forward 10 times.

This was: Easy   Slightly Challenging   Hard

Turn a full circle (360 degrees) taking only 4 steps.

This was: Easy   Slightly Challenging   Hard

- If you circled 6 Easy, you probably have GREAT balance. Congratulations! Use this book to learn how your balance system works so you can keep your balance in excellent condition.
- If you circled 5 Easy, you probably have GOOD balance. Not bad! Use this book to learn how to make your balancing ability great!
- If you circled 4 or fewer Easy, you probably need to work on your balance. Use this book to help you improve your balance gently and safely.

Now that you've assessed your balance, you must learn how to challenge yourself to move beyond your limits. Each time you reach outside of your balance safety zone, you have challenged your limits and done a balance exercise.

Balance is like a muscle; it responds well to exercise. Everyone can improve their balance, no matter how fit or frail you feel. With balance, there is always room for improvement.

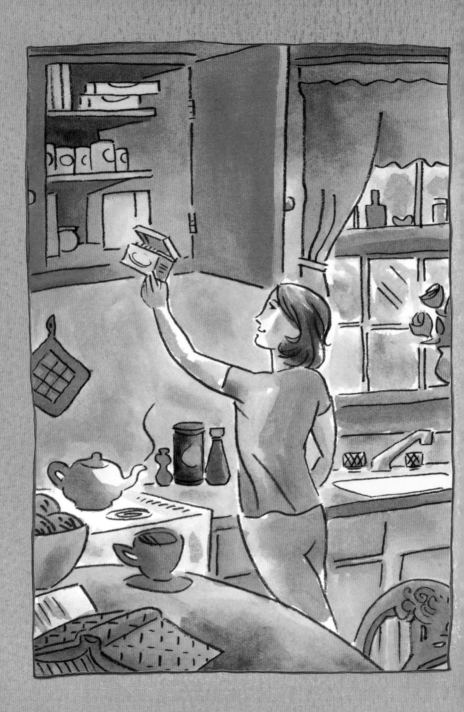

The Balance Routine

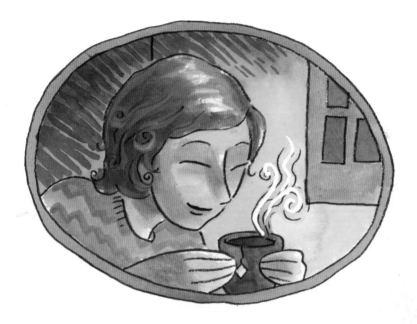

The balance training exercises in this routine are designed to increase your strength, stability, and flexibility. The routine begins with simple exercises and gradually progresses to more advanced ones. This program is suitable for almost everyone of any age. It is always a good idea to talk to your doctor before starting any exercise program.

In the Extra Attention boxes, you will find suggestions to make each exercise easier or more challenging to suit your needs. The audio CD in the back of the book will lead you through the routine in about fifteen minutes. For best results, however, read the book first and get familiar with each exercise before using the CD.

You can perform this balance training program at any time of the day, but doing it before or after your morning cup will help you establish a healthy routine. When you first get out of bed, you might feel a bit stiff. Walk around the house for 2-3 minutes, or simply walk in place, pumping your arms to get your blood flowing. Warming up is always a good idea prior to exercising.

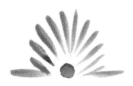

Follow these other tips for best results:

- Wear loose, comfortable clothing that allows you to move freely. Consider performing the exercises barefooted to allow you to feel your feet and ankles and help you develop your kinesthetic awareness.

- If your floors are dusty or wet, they can be slippery! Go barefoot only when you are sure that your floor can provide good traction and is free of anything that might cut or injure your feet.

- If you wear shoes, make sure they fit comfortably and provide adequate traction. Your foot should NOT slide inside of the shoe or feel like it is about to come off. No sandals or high heels! A comfortable walking or athletic shoe is best.

- Sit down and rest if you feel dizzy or lightheaded. Do not continue with the program until these feelings pass. If they don't pass within a couple of minutes, consult your doctor.

- Exercise should never cause pain. If a movement is painful, stop doing it. Try making the movement slower and/or smaller. If that doesn't help, skip to the next exercise.

- Keep your breath natural and relaxed during the routine. Listening to your body's natural rhythm of breath has a very calming effect on your central nervous system. Whenever possible, breathe in and out through your nose and relax your lower abdomen to allow deeper breathing. Never hold or restrict your breathing.

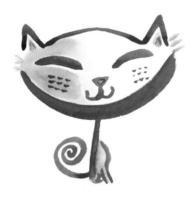

Eye Exercises

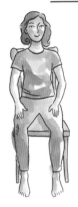

Your vision is very important to maintaining balance. Weak eye muscles can make your vision jerky, which in turn can make you feel unsteady. Smooth eyes movements will make you feel more stable.

Up - Down

1. Sit in a chair, hands on thighs, looking straight ahead.

2. Without moving your head, look up at the ceiling. As your eyes move up, imagine that you are tracking a slow rocket ship blasting off.

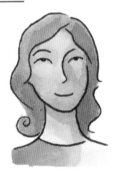

3. Now move your eyes down to the floor. As your eyes move down, imagine that you are tracking a balloon floating to the floor. Don't move your head, just your eyes.

4. Repeat five times.

Right - Left

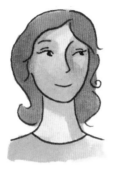

1. Without moving your head, look as far as you can to the RIGHT and then as far as you can to the LEFT.

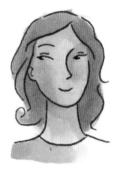

2. As your eyes move from side to side, imagine that you are tracking a bird flying across the horizon.

3. Repeat five times.

Extra Attention

You might experience slight dizziness with this exercise. If you do, make your eye movement slower, and pause briefly between each repetition. To exercise your visual acuity, let your gaze zero in on something specific as you reach the end point of your gaze up, down, right, and left. Sharpen your focus as if you were an eagle looking for something to eat.

Head Circles

Studies have shown that tense, rigid neck muscles can interfere with balance. This exercise will help you relax your neck and upper shoulders.

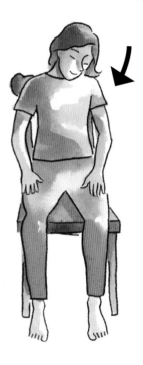

1. Without moving your body, slowly rotate your head as if you were drawing circles with your nose.

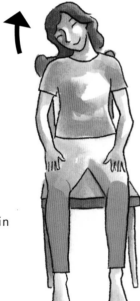

2. Circle five times in each direction.

3. Allow your breath and movement to be smooth and relaxed. Make the circles as large as you comfortably can. Listen to your body.

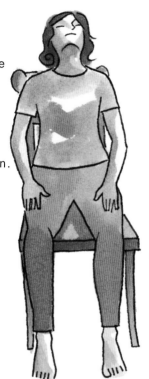

4. Learn to avoid movements that cause pain. In time, your muscles will relax and your movements will get larger. Be patient.

Extra Attention

Head movements stimulate your inner ear/vestibular system. You might experience slight dizziness with this exercise. If you do, make your head circles smaller and slower. Give yourself time to recover from each rotation. With practice, your inner ear will get used to the activity, and you will not feel as dizzy.

Sit to Stand

Standardized balance tests often measure your ability to come to a standing position using your leg strength only. This skill measures strength and flexibility of the lower body, which are needed to maintain balance.

1. Sit on the edge of a firm, stable chair with your knees bent to get your feet flat and under you.

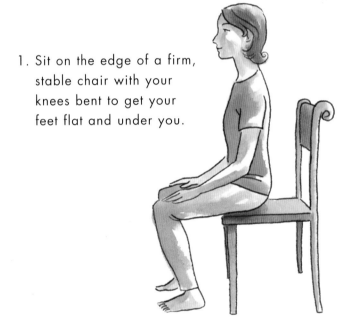

Extra Attention

To make this exercise easier, use your arms to assist you as much as you need, either by your side or using them for leverage. To make it more challenging, move slower, even pausing at the halfway spot.

2. Bend and reach forward
   with your arms, slowly
   rising to a full
   standing position.
   Do your best to keep
   your knees separated.

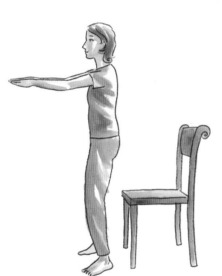

3. Return to your seat
   by slowly lowering
   yourself. This is a
   controlled movement.
   Do your best to avoid
   plopping.

4. Repeat five times.

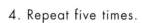

Standing to the Four

Standing to the Four is an ancient Chinese exercise designed to help you balance your body weight equally through your feet. A balanced standing posture provides stability.

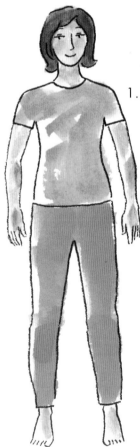

1. Stand with your feet shoulder width apart and parallel.

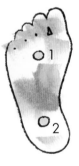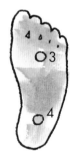

2. Imagine four points on the bottom of your feet.

3. Keeping your feet flat on the floor, gently rock forward and back to identify the points under the balls of your feet and centers of your heels.

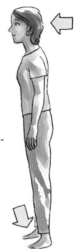

4. Keeping your feet flat on the floor, gently rock side-to-side to identify the two points under your right foot and the two points under your left foot.

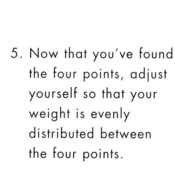

5. Now that you've found the four points, adjust yourself so that your weight is evenly distributed between the four points.

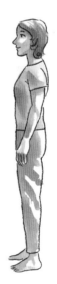

6. Maintain your Standing to the Four posture for one minute.

Standing to the Three

Standing to the Three is an ancient Chinese exercise designed to help you align your posture vertically. A tall upright posture provides stability.

1. Stand with your feet flat, shoulder width apart and parallel.

2. Imagine that your body is made up of three spheres, like a snowman.

3. Using your imagination as your guide, stack your three spheres directly on top of the other. Gently focus on the imagery. Your bodymind will strive to correct any imbalances that exist. You will develop a sense of being vertically balanced and upright.

4. Maintain your Standing to the Three posture for one minute.

These are examples of not properly Standing to the Three:

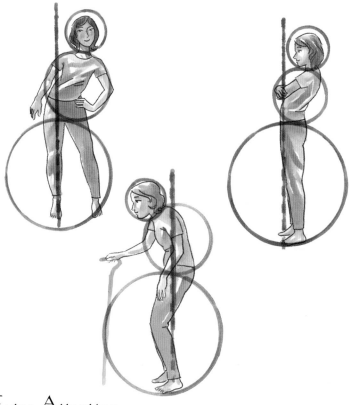

Extra Attention

Using imagery to guide your posture is a skill that gets better with practice. Soon, your ability to sense and correct your postural alignment will improve dramatically. Take the next step and combine Standing to the Four and Standing to the Three. Gently balance the imagery of the two exercises and maintain standing quietly for a total of two minutes.

Counter Swing

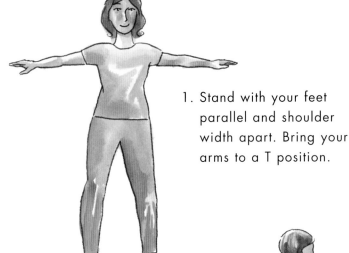

1. Stand with your feet parallel and shoulder width apart. Bring your arms to a T position.

2. Drop your arms, and twist to your left. The twist occurs primarily at your waist. Keep your hips and knees pointing forward.

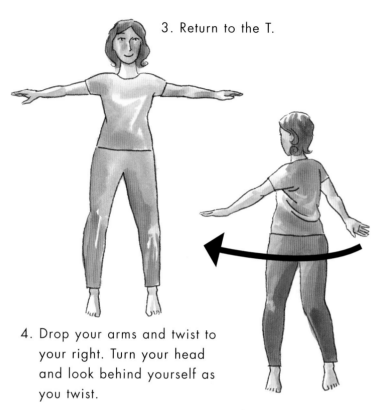

3. Return to the T.

4. Drop your arms and twist to your right. Turn your head and look behind yourself as you twist.

5. Continue alternating your twist left and right for a count of ten.

Extra Attention

Your ability to twist or rotate is key to maintaining balance. You need a supple spine to move freely and change direction at will. Remember to keep your hips and knees pointing forward so you're focusing on rotating your spine. Spinal rotation tends to decrease with age, but this simple exercise will help keep your neck and spine mobile.

Rise and Drop

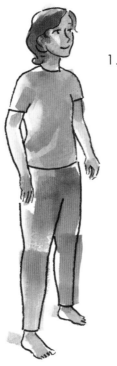

1. Stand with your feet parallel and shoulder width apart.

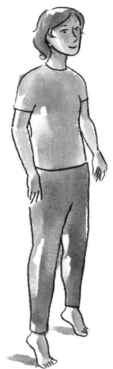

2. Slowly shift your weight to the balls of your feet and lift your heels off the floor.

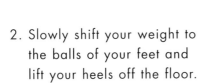

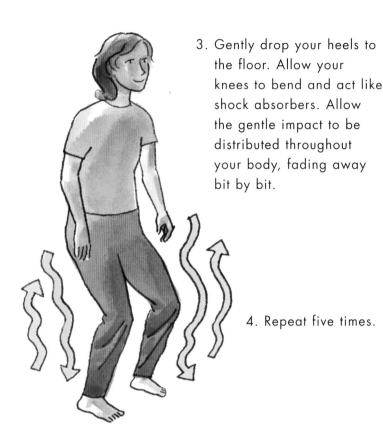

3. Gently drop your heels to the floor. Allow your knees to bend and act like shock absorbers. Allow the gentle impact to be distributed throughout your body, fading away bit by bit.

4. Repeat five times.

Extra Attention

When you are stiff, an impact will knock you off balance. When you are resilient, an impact will jostle you, but you can remain in control. This exercise will teach you how to absorb bumps and jostles. It also builds strength and flexibility in your feet, ankles, and lower legs.

Trembling Horse

This ancient Chinese exercise is modeled on a horse shaking its skin to get rid of a fly. You may be more familiar with the image of a wet dog shaking water off his back. Think of how the rippling motion moves from the dog's head, all the way down, until it reaches the tip of his tail.

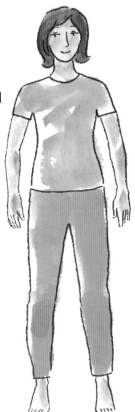

1. Stand with your feet parallel and shoulder width apart. Inhale.

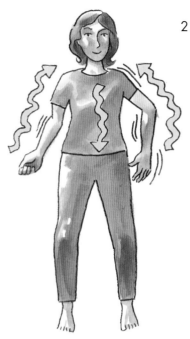

2. As you exhale, gently wiggle your fingers, then your elbows, shoulders, ribcage, hips, knees, ankles, and finally your feet.

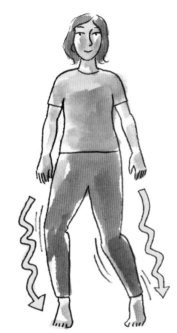

3. Repeat 5 times.

Extra Attention

Think of this exercise as a total body scan. Notice what feels wiggly and what feels stiff. You are developing your kinesthetic awareness. Do not force the stiff areas to wiggle. Take a mental note; for example, tell yourself, "My hips feel stiff." In time, your body will feel like a healthy tree bending and blowing in the wind.

Spiral Low-High

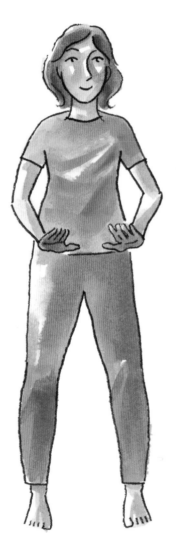

1. Stand with your feet parallel and shoulder width apart. Place your hands in front of you.

2. Move your hands in a clockwise circle, starting with a small, tight circle, then spiraling out larger and larger until you are reaching as high and as low as your limits allow.

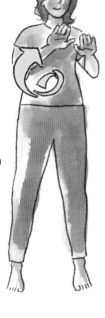

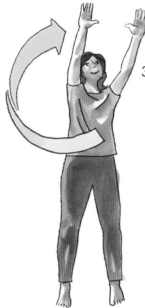

3. Change direction and spiral inward to your starting position. Move slowly. Keep your feet flat on the floor.

Extra Attention

AWARENESS. Although this exercise will build your strength and flexibility, put your attention on the sensations that you are feeling. It is easy to feel your arms working, but try shifting your attention lower. Feel the weight of your body as it travels across the bottoms of your feet. Remember the four points from page 32?

Side-to-Side Reach

The distance you can reach is often measured to assess balance. Lateral reaching, or reaching to the side, requires strength and stability in your torso, legs, and shoulders.

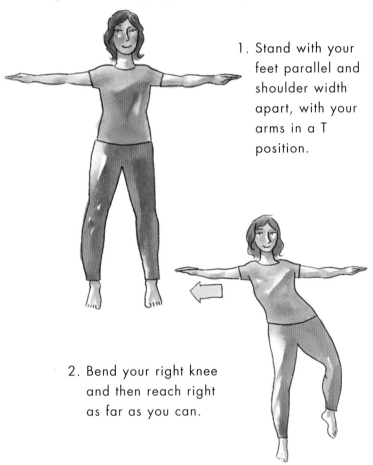

1. Stand with your feet parallel and shoulder width apart, with your arms in a T position.

2. Bend your right knee and then reach right as far as you can.

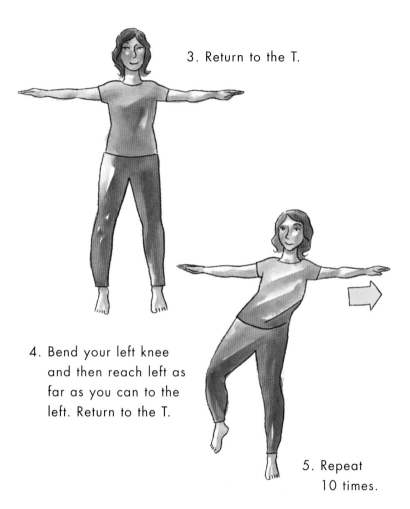

3. Return to the T.

4. Bend your left knee and then reach left as far as you can to the left. Return to the T.

5. Repeat 10 times.

Extra Attention

It is okay to lift your opposite foot off of the floor to increase your reach distance. Pay attention to your limits and listen to your body!

Polishing the Table

This exercise can be done with or without a table. If using a table, be sure not to lean against the table or use it for support.

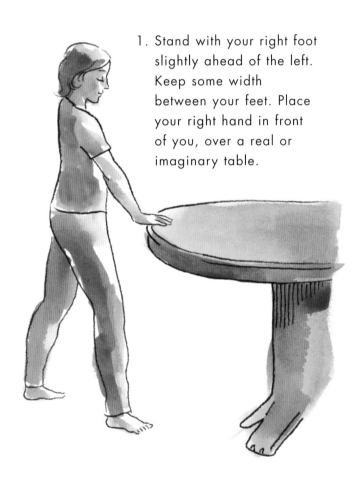

1. Stand with your right foot slightly ahead of the left. Keep some width between your feet. Place your right hand in front of you, over a real or imaginary table.

2. Move your hand in a clockwise circle, spiraling out larger and larger until you are reaching as far as your limits allow.

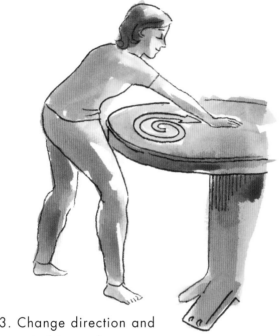

3. Change direction and spiral inward to your starting position.

4. Repeat with left foot forward using your left hand.

Extra Attention

Do not allow your knee to extend past your toe as you are reaching forward. Gently focus on the sensations that you feel as you shift your weight forward to extend your reach. Can you feel the muscles working? Are you challenging your balance safety zone?

Fast-Stepping Drill

1. Quickly, take 4 steps forward, right-left-right-left, then freeze!

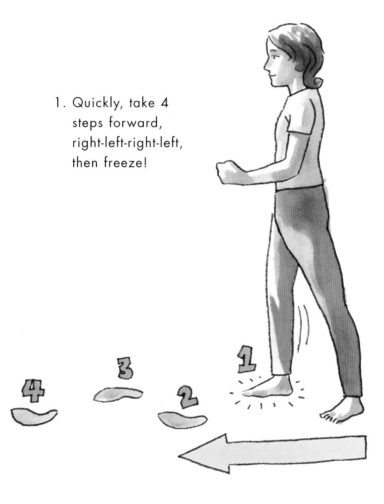

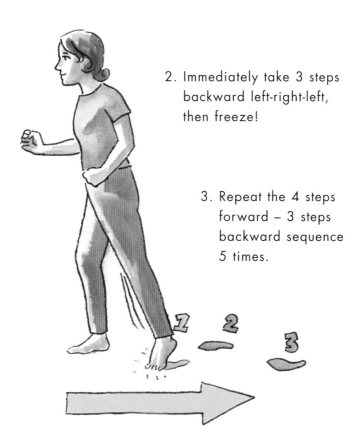

2. Immediately take 3 steps backward left-right-left, then freeze!

3. Repeat the 4 steps forward – 3 steps backward sequence 5 times.

Extra Attention

Changing direction quickly requires agility—the combination of strength, balance, and coordination. Challenge yourself to move as quickly as your balance allows. Be in charge of your momentum. Learn to "put on the brakes" and "throw it in reverse." Stay in control.

Slow-Stepping Drill

Maintaining control of your body while moving slowly requires an extreme amount of strength and balance. Challenge yourself to move as slowly as you can.

Slow Motion Step Forward

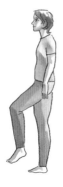

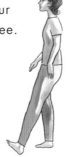

1. Lift your left knee.

2. Gently place your left heel on the floor.

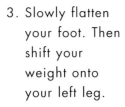

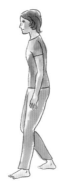

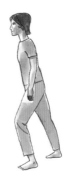

3. Slowly flatten your foot. Then shift your weight onto your left leg.

4. Take 3 more steps forward, right, left, right.

Slow Motion Step Backward

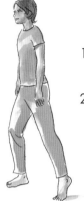

1. Lift your left knee.

2. Gently place your left toe on the floor behind you.

3. Slowly flatten your left foot, then shift your weight onto your left leg.

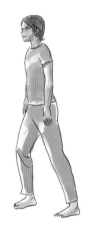

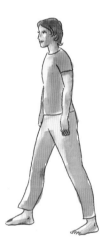

4. Take 3 more steps back.

Extra Attention

Pay attention to the details of each movement. How high can you lift your knee? How gently can you place your heel/toe on the floor? How slowly can you shift your weight on to your foot? In essence, you are practicing Tai Chi stepping. Learn more about Tai Chi on page 67.

Side-Stepping Drill

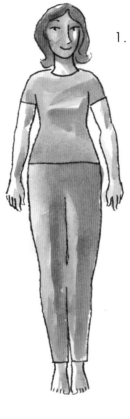

1. Begin with your feet together, knees slightly bent.

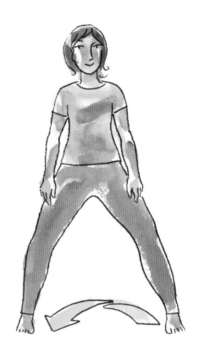

2. Keeping your left knee bent, lift your right foot and step as wide as you comfortably can.

3. Slightly bend
   your right knee
   and slide your
   left foot in.

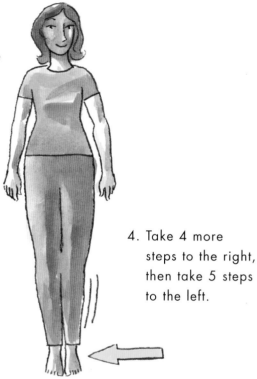

4. Take 4 more
   steps to the right,
   then take 5 steps
   to the left.

Extra Attention

Challenge yourself by varying your speed. Take several steps in slow motion like the previous exercise. Then take a few more steps, moving quickly. Take mental notes on what your body feels like when you are moving slowly, and when you are moving quickly. Pay attention to being in control of the movement. Take charge of your momentum.

Walking a Figure 8

Visualizing your path before you walk it will bring focus and clarity to your movement.

1. Place one chair several feet directly in front of another. Stand behind the first chair, turn to your right or left, then walk a path between the chairs in the shape of the numeral 8.

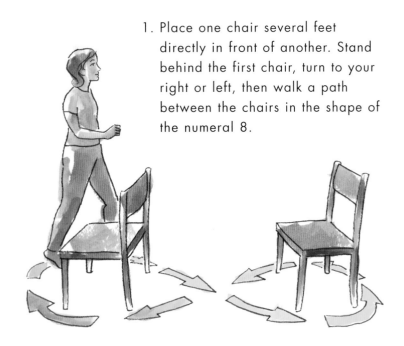

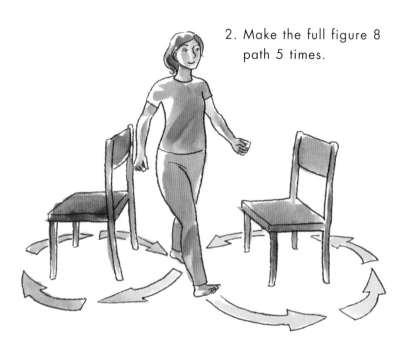

2. Make the full figure 8
path 5 times.

Extra Attention

Challenge yourself by varying your speed. Try walking very, very
slow. Try walking very, very fast. Challenge yourself even more by
removing the chairs and making the Figure 8 very small. The tighter
the turns, the harder it is to keep your balance!

Ball Toss

If you don't have a ball at home, pick one up the next time you go to the grocery store or use a small pillow.

1. Stand with your feet parallel and shoulder width apart, and hold a ball with both hands.

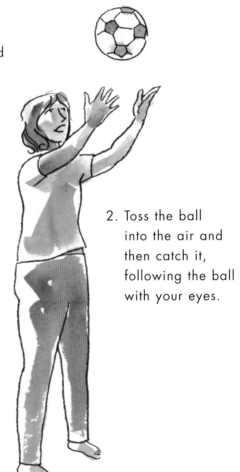

2. Toss the ball into the air and then catch it, following the ball with your eyes.

3. Repeat 5 times.

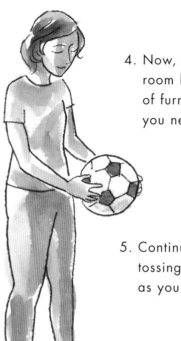

4. Now, begin walking around the room holding the ball. Take note of furniture and obstacles that you need to avoid.

5. Continue walking, and start tossing and catching the ball as you walk.

6. Repeat for 10-15 throws.

Extra Attention

Walking and playing catch simultaneously can feel like patting your head and rubbing your tummy. It requires dividing your attention among several tasks. Multi-tasking is a skill that tends to diminish with age. You can increase the cognitive demands of this exercise by combining it with your other stepping drills: Slow, Fast, Sideways, and Figure 8.

Bend and Reach

1. Stand with your hands on your hips, right foot slightly ahead of the left. Keep some width between your feet.

2. Bend your right knee and reach toward the floor as far as you comfortably can.

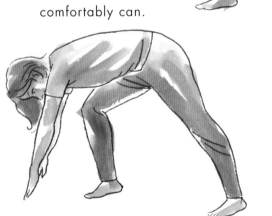

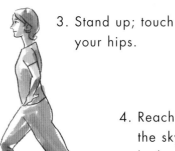

3. Stand up; touch your hips.

4. Reach toward the sky and look upwards.

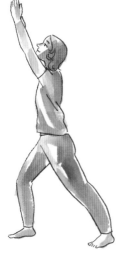

5. Return your hands to your hips. Repeat 4 times.

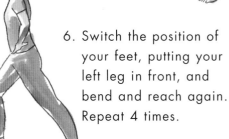

6. Switch the position of your feet, putting your left leg in front, and bend and reach again. Repeat 4 times.

Extra Attention

Pay close attention to your knee as you reach for the floor. Do not allow your knee to extend past your toes as it causes undue stress and strain. Bending requires strength and flexibility in the spine, hips, and legs. Do not force your movement. Pay attention to your limits and progress at your own pace.

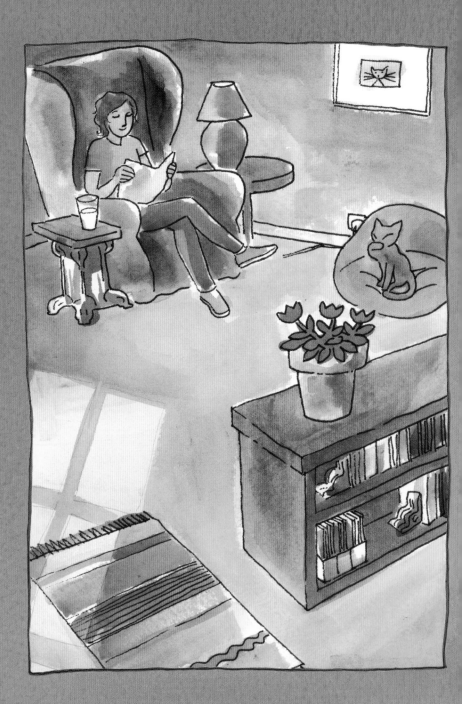

Getting the Most from Your Balance Routine

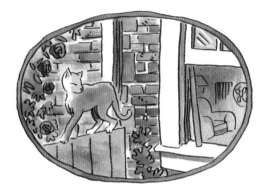

Take a breath, and enjoy your new, less cluttered surroundings and your increased balance, strength, and flexibility. Feel free to practice any or all of your balance routine throughout the day.

For best results, do the routine 3-5 times each week. You should notice an improvement in your balance in as little as two weeks.

The next two sections offer some extra balance exercises, and combining one or both with your balance routine will help you get the most out of your routine and everyday life.

Not all falls can be prevented, but now you have the tools you need to reduce your risk of sustaining a fall-related injury. Be safe, be strong, be happy!

Using Imagery for Better Balance

Your body contains all of the information you need to know to stay happy and healthy. Your mission is to learn how to listen and respond to these signals.

The New Forest 1 through 10 imagery was created by John Bright-Fey to help Tai Chi and meditation students focus mind and body on coordinated, regenerative physical activity. When your body and mind work together as they should, you enter what John calls "The New Forest." I have applied his system to balance training. Your brain and body, or bodymind, respond well to the language of imagination and imagery. The New Forest 1 through 10 imagery provides you with a kind of vocabulary so you can communicate with your bodymind.

Start by reading the following list aloud several times.

NUMBER	KEYWORD
1	FUN
2	SHOE
3	TREE
4	CORE
5	ALIVE
6	THICK
7	HEAVEN
8	GATE
9	SHINE
10	SPIN

Now, close your eyes and count from one through ten, saying the numbers and keywords from memory. Recite silently or aloud; you choose. If you get stuck, open your eyes and read the list again until you know all of the keywords and their associated numbers. It won't be long before you have them easily memorized. Each keyword provides a concept and bodymind skill that will help you relate to and improve your balance.

You can think about any or all of these as you go through your balance routine, or use the 1 to 10 imagery by itself any time you need more balance.

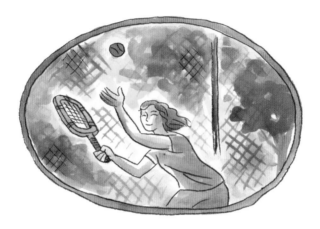

1-FUN

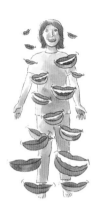

Think of fun. Smile gently and suggest to yourself to relax all over. Tension impairs your ability to sense and respond to changes in your body and in your environment.

QUESTION: Do I feel relaxed, or am I holding my muscles tense and rigid?

2-SHOE

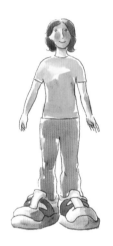

Think about your toes, feet, and the shoes you're usually wearing standing firmly on the ground. Be alert to changes in terrain that might affect how your feet connect you to the earth.

QUESTION: Can I feel the floor through the bottoms of my feet?

3-TREE

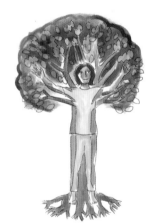

Imagine that you are a healthy tree with roots penetrating deeply into the soil. You are rooted, vibrant, and stable. You can move and sway in the wind without falling.

QUESTION: Do I feel rooted to the earth like a big tree?

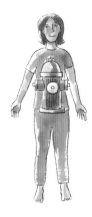

4-CORE

Imagine that you have a fire hydrant buried deep inside your abdomen. This is your "core" or physical center of gravity. Controlling your center gives you confidence in your movements.

QUESTION: Can I feel my center of gravity deep inside my belly?

5-ALIVE

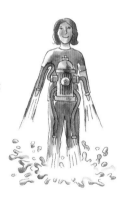

Pretend that pressurized life-giving water from your 4-CORE is rushing out of your arms and legs at an incredible speed. Suggest to yourself that all movement begins at your 4-CORE. Your arms and legs are connected to and get their strength from your center.

QUESTION: Am I paying attention to how I move my arms and legs?

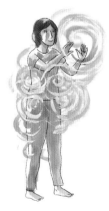

6-THICK

Pretend that all of the air around you is thick and viscous. The thick air connects you to your surroundings. Through it you can feel the stationary and moving objects that might become an obstacle and affect your stability.

QUESTION: Am I aware of what is around me?

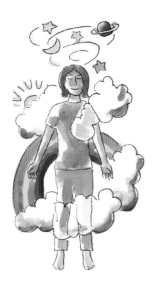

7-HEAVEN

Gently stretch up with the top of your head toward the heavens as if you were a marionette. Pretend that an imaginary thread is subtly lifting you upward, guiding you to stand straight and tall.

QUESTION: Do I need to stand taller and stop slouching?

8-GATE

Imagine that each pore of your skin is in reality a tiny gate. As you inhale, these gates open; as you exhale, these gates close. Feeling off-balance can cause you to hold or restrict your breathing. Pretend that you are breathing with every inch of your skin.

QUESTION: Am I taking full deep breaths?

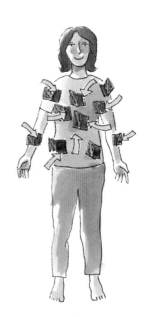

9-SHINE

Imagine that you are a light bulb. As you inhale, your light is dim. As you exhale, you shine out brighter and brighter. Depression, anger, and fear impair your emotional and physical balance. Project a positive attitude like a light shining brightly. Exert yourself evenly in all directions.

QUESTION: Do I have a positive attitude about my balance?

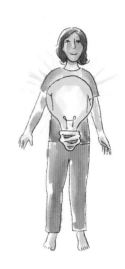

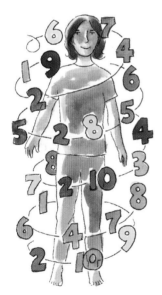

10-SPIN

Let the first 9 numbers and their associated images float through your mind in any order. If one pops in your mind with more clarity than the others, focus on it briefly, and then let it slip away until another comes up. Mental and physical flexibility is crucial to maintaining balance.

QUESTION: Am I giving myself permission to do things differently?

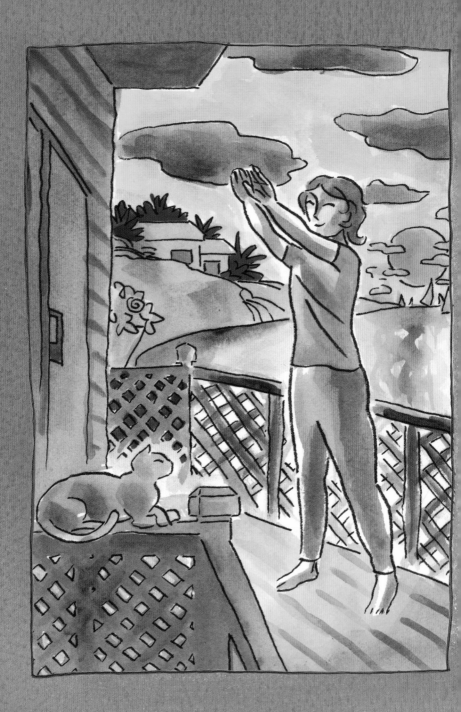

A Sip of Tai Chi for Balance

I couldn't write a book on balance exercises without teaching you a little Tai Chi. Tai Chi ("tie chee") is a form of exercise that was created in China more than 1,000 years ago. Today, it is recognized as one of the most effective balance training systems in existence. Medical research indicates that the regular practice of Tai Chi can reduce the chances that an older adult will fall by nearly 50 percent.

For your extra sip, I will introduce you to a very simple version of New Forest Tai Chi, a modern style created to make the health benefits of Tai Chi available to everyone. Compared to traditional styles of Tai Chi, New Forest Tai Chi is very easy to learn. There are no confusing postures or complicated movements. It is Tai Chi for people just like you.

New Forest Tai Chi is presented in detail in *A Morning Cup of Tai Chi* by John Bright-Fey. The book tells you a lot about the history, philosophy, and technique of Tai Chi. I highly recommend it! But for now, why don't you take a sip and try a simplified form of New Forest Tai Chi.

When stepping forward and backward in the exercises on the next pages, you'll use basic Tai Chi stepping. The lifting of your knee, the placing of your foot, and the gradual shifting of your body weight is slow and deliberate.

Incorporate the imagery associated with each number from the previous pages.

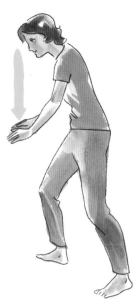

1. Take a slow motion step forward with your right foot. Keeping both feet flat on the floor, lift both arms as high as comfortable and paint a large number 1. Remember, the key word is fun.

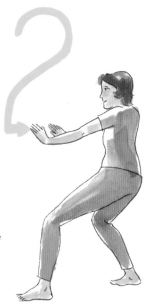

2. Take a slow motion step forward with your left foot. Plant both feet flat. Lift your arms, slowly. Paint the shape of a number 2 in slow motion. Remember, the key word is shoe.

3. Step forward again, remembering to move as slowly as possible. Paint a number 3.

   Allow your torso to twist to the right and left. Imagine that you are a tree with deep roots, swaying in the wind. Remember, the key word is tree.

4. Take another slow motion step forward, plant your feet, and slowly paint the number 4. Feel the heaviness of your center. Remember, the key word is core.

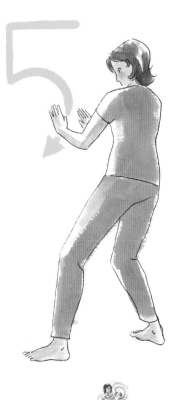

5. One more time, step forward, slowly. Lift your arms and paint the number 5. Move slowly. Feel yourself reach, twist, turn, and shift. Remember, the key word is alive.

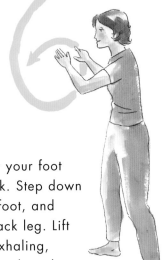

6. Now, change direction. Lift your foot slowly and take a step back. Step down with your toe, flatten your foot, and shift your weight to your back leg. Lift your arms as you inhale. Exhaling, draw a big number 6. Remember, the key word is thick.

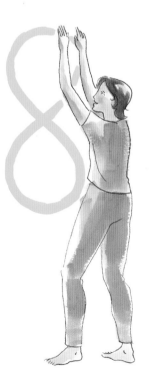

7. Take another slow motion step backward. Plant both feet flat. Lift your arms, slowly. Paint the shape of a number 7 in slow motion. Remember, the key word is heaven.

8. Step back again, remembering to move as slowly as possible. Paint a number 8.

Eights are curvy. Allow your torso to twist to the right and left. Remember, the key word is gate.

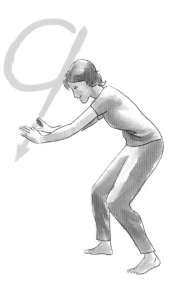

9. Take another slow motion step backward, plant your feet, and slowly paint the number 9. Remember, the key word is shine.

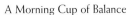

10. One more time, step back, slowly. Lift your arms and paint the number 10. You can paint the number 1 followed by the number 0 or you can let your left hand make the 1 and your right hand make the 0. Remember, the key word is spin.

Tips for Preventing Falls

Wear the right shoes. Shoes should be: ～～～

- Easy to tie and have strings that aren't too long
- Flat-soled – high heels can cause balance problems
- Non-skid with a wide base
- Comfortable and fit properly

Don't: ～～～

- Drink too much alcohol
- Walk on surfaces that are uneven or sloping
- Walk on wet or slippery surfaces
- Walk in places that do not have proper lighting
- Walk while wearing glasses that make you dizzy – bifocals can be especially risky
- Go up or down stairways that are dark or don't have handrails

Do: ～～～

- Exercise – balance-building exercises like Tai Chi, as well as strengthening exercises can improve your balance and help you avoid falls
- Be aware if you are taking medication that makes you dizzy
- Avoid slippery surfaces such as tile or hardwood floors that have recently been waxed
- Use non-slip mats in the bath tub and shower surfaces
- Remove tripping hazards from your home and avoid them when out of the home
- Make sure stairwells have hand rails on both sides
- Install grab bars in the bathroom next to the bath tub and toilet and in the shower

If you would like to learn more about...

<u>KIM BRIGHT-FEY, PT</u> – Author of *A Morning Cup of Balance*
www.ImproveYourBalance.com

<u>NEW FOREST TAI CHI</u> – Lessons, Books, DVDs
www.NewForestWay.com

<u>BALANCE DISORDERS</u>
1. National Institute on Deafness and Other
   Communication Disorders
   National Institutes of Health
   www.nidcd.nih.gov/health/balance/index.asp

2. American Physical Therapy Association
   www.apta.org

<u>PREVENTING FALLS</u>
National Center for Injury Prevention and Control
www.cdc.gov

<u>BOOKS AND DVDs BY KIM BRIGHT-FEY:</u>
1. *A Morning Cup of Massage:* one 15-minute routine for a
   lifetime of energy & harmony

2. New Forest Tai Chi for Beginners DVD
   UPC: 827912001556

The Morning Cup™ Series

If you want other exercises to improve your balance, try:

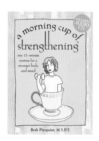 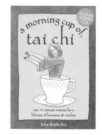 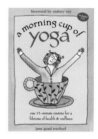

To increase your strengthening and flexibility:

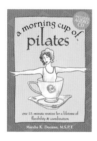 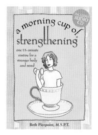 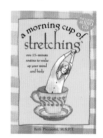

To increase your energy and well-being:

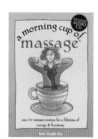 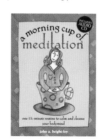 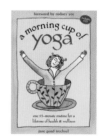

About the Author

Kim Bright-Fey is a licensed physical therapist who is certified with the American Physical Therapy Association as a health and wellness consultant. She has been teaching Qigong, Tai Chi, and therapeutic exercise since 1988. She lives in Birmingham, Alabama.

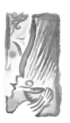

Routine at a Glance

Eye Exercises

Head Circles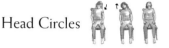

Sit to Stand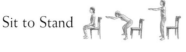

Standing to the Four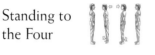

Standing to the Three

Counter Swing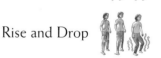

Rise and Drop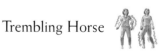

Trembling Horse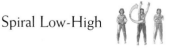

Spiral Low-High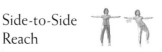

Side-to-Side Reach

Polishing the Table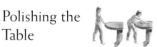

Fast-Stepping Drill

Slow Stepping Drill

Side Stepping Drill

Walking a Figure 8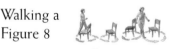

Ball Toss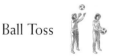

Bend and Reach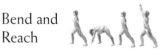

Tear this page out and post it on your refrigerator or another handy spot for quick reference to your balance routine.

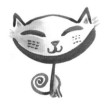